More Than
A
Speed Bump

More Than A Speed Bump
©2012 Jim Scott

Published by RiverRun Select
An imprint of Piscataqua Press and
RiverRun Bookstore
142 Fleet St
Portsmouth, NH 03801

info@riverrunbookstore.com
www.riverrunbookstore.com
www.piscataquapress.com

ISBN: 978-0-9885370-7-1

Printed in the United States of America

More than a Speed Bump

Life before and after
a Traumatic Brain Injury

By Jim Scott

Acknowledgements

I am grateful to so many people who have played a vital and important role in my life. There are so many that I simply cannot mention them all in my story, but these wonderful individuals from teachers, athletic coaches, doctors, volunteers, interns, the incredibly inspiring brain injury survivors I've met at The Krempels' Center (KC) and KC's staff, have provided me with the strength that comes from the knowledge that I'm never alone. My deepest thanks go to Ted King for his encouragement and the introduction to post-TBI competitive sports. For your constant support, encouragement, and belief in me, thank you Barry Dyke. Of course, thank you to my unconditionally loving, supportive family and great friends. Thanks to Rachel Forrest, for helping me put this book together. Last but not least, Boomer, thank you for 14 years and 1 month of loyal companionship.

One Night That Changed Everything

It was July 3, 2006 and like many people my age—23-I was gearing up for a week of holiday partying. My family had moved to Maine, with most of my friends and the parties in my hometown, Atkinson, NH where I stayed at the home of my wonderful lifelong friends, the Reardons. Everything I know about what happened that night and during the weeks after, I know only from my mother's detailed notes and police reports. I have no other clear recollection but one last memory of washing my father's Mercedes SL55 with Mr. Reardon in his driveway.

On that night my friend Derek Reardon and I went to a bar in Atkinson to start drinking before we moved the partying to an old friend's house. I have no memory of being there, but for some odd reason I decided to drive home. This is still a mystery to me. I wasn't a habitual drunk driver, but that doesn't matter because I know now that one time is all it takes. In fact, Derek and I had even made a plan for him to drive us home to his house and because of our plan Derek had stopped drinking.

I took an unusual route which was also a mystery to me. After the party, I took side roads—probably Routes 125 and 108, although Routes I-495 to I-95 would have been a straight shot to my house. At around 3 a.m. the police say I fell asleep at the wheel, although I probably passed out because my blood alcohol content was so high. The legal level in NH is .08 and mine was much higher. The car went

1

off the road and I was ejected as I didn't have a seat belt on. The car was absolutely demolished and had I remained in the driver's seat, I would have been crushed. The only reason the accident was discovered was because I miraculously dragged my bloodied body back to the roadside and, fortunately, a passerby saw me and called the authorities. I was taken to Exeter Hospital, unconscious, bloody and with no idea how tough I'd made my life going forward or how my life had changed forever.

The Beginning

How I got to that hospital room and the journey I've had to take since then begins with a familiar story of teenage life, one with a good family and a not so good amount of partying. I grew up an incredibly fortunate child in Southern NH with a loving, supportive family and great friends. My father worked tirelessly to provide my younger brother, Andy, older sister Aimee and me with everything we needed and many things we just wanted. We grew up well educated in a life of privilege.

Along with that great upbringing was my alcoholism. I can trace it back to the first time I got drunk at fourteen. I was at a hotel with one of my best friends for my brother's hockey tournament and we hung out in my parent's room while they were at dinner. We took shots from their bottle of vodka. I spent the next eight years trying to replicate the feeling of that first buzz. As is true in most alcoholics' stories, it took more and more alcohol to reach the same buzz, a cycle that lead to my accident.

I graduated high school in 2001, a decent three sport athlete and fairly popular. School was an absolute joke to me. I barely did any work and had ridiculously bad attendance. I wanted to attend a good college, but with my poor academic record I knew I needed to do something more to achieve this so I attended a postgraduate year at Loomis Chaffee, a prestigious prep school in Connecticut, to better ready myself for college. I did well in part due to their strict rules and in part because I stopped my excessive partying, which allowed me to apply myself academically.

I had a good year both athletically and academically at Loomis Chaffee and got accepted into Boston University where I would major in Business Management and play for the golf team. I made the Dean's List and had a good fall semester for the golf team. Once again, things came easily for me. I didn't study at all or practice even remotely hard for golf. I did well despite my laziness, but college life at BU was so repetitive and boring, I decided to leave. I remember the conversation in which I told my father about leaving. It was December and I had just completed the last final exam of my first semester, freshman year. I stood on the sidewalk of Boston's Commonwealth Avenue waiting for my dad to pick me up for Winter Break.

As soon as I got in the car and we headed home he asked, "So how did you do?" A pretty mundane question for a father to ask his son at the completion of his son's first college semester, but my answer was anything but mundane. "Well, I'm not going back," I replied. He asked why and I simply said that college wasn't for me and I was going to get a job and work instead. Surprisingly, despite his shock he understood. When my semester grades arrived a week or so later both my parents were confused that after doing so well at BU, I was nonetheless disenchanted with college and resolute in my decision.

As soon as I got home I worked for my Uncle Donny as a construction laborer, quite a change from being a student at BU. The work was physically hard, but I preferred it to what I felt was a snobby academic environment at BU, plus I got to work my great friend Kevin: We had a good time despite the harsh Maine winter.

The holidays were a bit awkward because I had to explain why I had decided to leave BU to everyone I knew. Days turned into weeks and I seriously thought about my future, realizing I needed some sort of college degree because I didn't want to work a physically taxing job my whole life. My parents made it abundantly clear that I could either work full-time and support myself completely or return to school, but if I lived at home I had to pay rent of some sort. Faced with this choice, I enrolled in classes at a community college and continued to work until I could decide on a college to transfer into. Winter dragged on and I was bored as hell. It was the first winter I hadn't played hockey so I headed south to where I felt I could play college golf and earn a degree at the same time.

I looked around and was intrigued by The University of Tampa because it had a good business school and I was confident I could play for their golf team. Coincidently, my paternal grandparents winter in Naples, a town about 2 hours away from Tampa. In spring of 2003, I told my grandfather "Grampy", who I was named after, about my interest and he suggested I come down to work a trade show for his lab supply company with him, and we would also visit the campus. I headed to Naples then drove up to Tampa, worked the show, and saw the campus. I was very impressed with the campus and the business school facility.

My grandfather, a very loving and supportive guy, was also impressed, although mostly with the fact the school was 75% female. Three years later I still had girls coming up to me saying, "How's your Grandfather doing? He's so cute." The school was hosting a sorority cookout the day we visited and my Grandfather introduced "his single grandson" to a good number of the coeds. When I returned home from the trip I told my mom I had decided to apply and she was very supportive. All winter I continued to work construction while dreaming of the Florida sunshine. I sent my application in and was accepted. I would enroll the following fall as a 21-year-old second semester freshmen. I felt rather old, but was excited to start fresh. I worked construction that summer to save up money to bring to school with me that fall.

I flew down to Tampa that August with my parents and moved into a dorm. I had a roommate who seemed a bit odd and depressed. He left school not long into the year and I had a single until my friend Derek moved in. I had a great time playing golf and actually enjoyed my choice of major, economics. I'm not saying I'm a genius or anything, but college was incredibly easy for me. I'd usually just scan the syllabus and show up only on exam days or when a presentation was given. Somehow I managed a GPA in the high 3's as a "part-time" student of sorts. Once I showed up for an exam and the professor demanded to see my student ID because she didn't remember seeing me that semester. In fact, one professor demanded to know, "who I was taking the exam for," and only relented after checking my ID against the class roster. I know I would have learned more in college and would have enjoyed learning more if I'd applied myself, but I saw college as something that just needed to be completed.

I finished the year and headed home to work construction for my uncle for the summer. By this time I had accumulated enough credits to be a junior and returned to UT that fall. I had made some close friends so we got a four bedroom apartment on campus. If you have seen the movie "Animal House," you can appreciate what our apartment was like. That year I might as well as had only two classes —hops and barley. I partied like crazy, but somehow managed to hold down an internship with a private equity firm in St. Petersburg, while continuing to do well, actually just ok, athletically and academically. Everything was going well. It was that April that my idyllic life would be shattered.

"Is Andy going to live?"

On April 23, 2005, just fourteen months before my own horrific car crash, my brother Andy was in his own serious accident. He's younger by 4 years and we get along great. Sure, we've had the brotherly fights—some physical and some verbal—but he's not only my brother, he's my best friend. The great afternoons playing golf, home run derby battles in the back yard, and the times he made me stay out in the dark being attacked by mosquitoes so he could cast "just one more" fishing line in the lake are some of the happiest moments of my life.

Now, he was in trouble. At about 10 a.m. on April 24 I was still in bed nursing another all too familiar hangover when the phone rang. The memory of that phone call from my father about Andy's accident is still vivid.

"Jim," he began. "I just wanted to let you know that Andy had an accident in Mexico and I'm on my way to Houston where he has been airlifted. He's in rough shape, but I won't really know any more details until I arrive in Texas and talk to his doctors."

I sobbed when my father explained that after a night of partying, Andy fell from a 3rd story balcony at his hotel in Cancun. He was stable, but in rough shape. I was wrecked. I felt it was my job to protect my little brother so I felt like a complete loser and that I was somewhat responsible. In high school I had a reputation for being a heavy drinker and I was sure this only added to the pressure to fit in

7

through alcohol use for Andy that many high school kids face. "What does this mean? How bad is it?" I asked.

My father, who is very emotional about all his children, broke down in tears. He said he hadn't seen the doctor and couldn't say for sure, but that my mom, who had accompanied Andy to Cancun on the vacation, said he was about to have surgery on a broken vertebrae.

I was shocked and petrified. I knew anything spinal was very serious and demanded more details.

"Is Andy going to live?" I asked through my tears.

"Well the good news is that they have him stable, but I don't know how bad the damage is," my dad replied.

I demanded to fly to Houston from Tampa right away. My father tried to calm me down. He wanted to talk to the medical team before deciding on a plan for me so we decided that since I was in the midst of final exams, I would sit tight and wait for more information. As it was, my father had not even arrived in Houston yet.

I called my sister Aimee, who is a year older than I am and lived in California. She had just received a similar call and we were both crying. My sister has a way of soothing me no matter what the problem and I was at the point where she had to prevent me from getting in my car and driving to Houston right then. She calmed me down and I agreed that my parents really didn't need to have the additional worry of me dropping out of school and driving halfway across the country. We decided to wait until my dad said we should both come to Houston and meet there so the whole family could be together. I frantically emailed my professors explaining the situation and all of them were flexible and concerned. This was very comforting as I tried to manage my emotions.

My dad called me back and told me he had arrived in Houston and that Aimee and I should fly in the next morning. I coordinated a flight with Aimee so we would arrive at Houston's Hobby Airport at the same time. The whole experience is a blur, but I think it was a Monday when we both arrived in Houston, I from

Tampa and Aimee from San Francisco where she worked as a brand manager for the Clorox Company. Usually we would have been enthused to see one another, but this time, we were in tears. She had no idea at the time, but this would be the first of two cross-country trips that she would make within fifteen months to visit a badly injured brother.

We caught a cab and I asked the driver to bring us to St. Luke's Hospital, where Andy had been taken. Aimee had a wonderfully calming effect on me and by the time we arrived at the hospital we were more composed and decided we wanted be upbeat and positive when we faced what we both feared, our beloved brother lying in a hospital bed

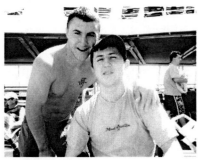

My brother and I on a cruise in March of 2006

with a serious injury. As we entered his hospital room we saw our parents in front of a young man under heavy morphine sedation and obviously in great pain. We all gathered in a huddled embrace as my father explained what the doctor's had told him.

"Andy's spinal cord is being pinched by a crushed vertebrae and swelling in the affected area, but the cord has not been severed," he explained. "Right now he is paralyzed from the waist down and has no sensation in the area, but the doctor hopes that when the swelling subsides, Andy will regain the use of his legs."

I clung to that hopeful possibility for a long time but my hopes were completely unrealistic. He hasn't regained the use or the feeling in his legs. I kept walking into his hospital room half expecting him to simply feel better and get out of that bed. Aimee, my father, and I had a hotel room across the street from Houston's Rice University as my mom was spending each night on a chair in Andy's room. I woke up early in the morning; unable to get back to sleep and I'd go out running on the school's campus. I ran for about

9

an hour each time, my thoughts preoccupied with Andy and his situation.

On one day I showered, changed and headed to Andy's room determined to be upbeat when I saw him. I passed my dad, who was sitting in the hotel lobby after returning from a morning visit with Andy. I sat next to my dad on the couch and he tearfully told me that he had just spoken with a doctor who had told him, "Despite Andy's injury, Andy will one day be able to have children through modern medicine."

This fact about the possibility of reproduction requiring some sort of advanced medical procedure forced my father and I to realize the severity of the situation. I had to face the fact that Andy wouldn't simply feel better and suddenly be fine. I began to cry as well. At that exact moment, my sister walked into the lobby and as she often does, supported both of us. As my father shared the information he had just told me with her, Aimee quickly had a positive spin on the news.

"So he'll be able to have a kid, that's awesome," she said.

I hadn't thought of the news this way and couldn't have the wonderful appreciation for the positives that Aimee did. In reality, Andy could easily have died but he was alive, and that couldn't be taken for granted. It is this uncanny ability to recognize the positives of any situation that I greatly admire about Aimee. That night the three of us went out to dinner, my mom refusing to leave Andy's side. At dinner the reality that both Aimee and I had been ignoring came up. We both had to return to our worlds, which despite our traumatic trips to Houston, kept in motion.

Aimee had work and I had finals waiting. We made a tentative plan to return to our lives the following day but we both hated to have to leave. At this point my mom was staying in the hotel and that last night I snuck back to Andy's hospital room around midnight. Andy was asleep so I quietly crept in and went to the end of the bed where his feet were and gently grabbed his ankles praying for God to take the feeling from my arms and give it to Andy's legs.

No matter how hard I prayed nothing happened so I also offered my body as a trade to God. I prayed for God to put me in the hospital bed instead of Andy. I didn't know then that in a weird way this prayer would be answered in a little over than a year. I returned to the hotel and fell asleep. In the morning, Aimee and I said emotional goodbyes to both Andy and my parents then headed to the airport. Our flights left about the same time which was a blessing because had Aimee not been there to prop me up I would not have been able to leave.

When I returned to campus, I couldn't focus. I called my mom constantly for updates. That week was torture as I attempted to take my exams while in constant contact with my mother in Houston, but I somehow managed to finish off the year and booked a flight home. All of the details of my return home that summer are fuzzy, but I'm pretty sure my brother and parents made the flight from Houston to Boston prior to my flight from Tampa to Manchester, NH. My parents maxed out their credit cards to charter a med flight to Boston because the insurance company would only cover a commercial flight which Andy was in no condition to take. Andy would spend over a month at Boston's wonderful Spaulding Rehabilitation Hospital, beginning a strong connection between the hospital and the Scott family, a connection that would come up again in less than a year and a half.

My friend Kevin picked me up at the airport and was very supportive. I have an incredible friend in Kevin who has been like a brother since eighth grade, providing a constant positive force on my often self-destructive behavior. I cried as I told him of how scary my time in Houston had been. He let me know that he was there to do anything I needed and that everything would be O.K.

Andy settled into the rehabilitation phase of his recovery amazingly well. Throughout Andy's long stay at Spaulding my family and Andy's friends were incredible. Hardly a minute of any day passed without a visitor. I usually visited at night since Andy and his buddies turned the hospital's visiting area into a poker room during the day. I liked spending the evenings alone with Andy

11

watching DVD's and talking about how my summer golf tournaments were going. I tried to keep our conversations light and didn't ask him for details about the accident.

Many people left a lasting impression on me that summer through their unbelievable compassion towards my family. One great guy in particular was there every time I went in around lunch time. Mike Hill, the husband of one of both Andy's and my elementary school teachers, works near Boston and often brought subs and had lunch with Andy. This pattern of kindness would repeat itself when Mike often visited me at Spaulding. Andy worked hard with the goal of being home by his June graduation. My amazing mother also worked hard. Not only did she support Andy and act as a pillar of strength for our family, but she was also in the role of general contractor for the construction of our new home in Cape Neddick, Maine. It turned out to be good fortune that the construction wasn't completed so my mom could add an elevator to the plan when we realized Andy would probably be in a wheelchair when we moved into the house. Eventually and unbelievably, both of her sons would need the elevator to access the different levels of the house due to serious injuries.

Andy did come home for graduation. His classmates and their families gave him a standing ovation as he received his diploma. We hadn't yet moved into our new house with the elevator, so Andy had to be carried up the stairs to his bedroom each night. Although I was quite aware of the dangers of alcohol especially after my own brother's paralysis, I continued my excessive partying. I'd come home after a night of heavy drinking and somehow carry Andy up the stairs. I am ashamed to say that Andy had to stiff arm a few walls as I made my way down the hallway with him in my arms. I'm absolutely disgusted by the horrible example I set and how dangerous my behavior remained even after his accident. There's that cliché that says kids think they are invincible, but I have first-hand knowledge that it's quite true. I watched as alcohol use nearly caused the death of my own brother, yet I continued to party and drink dangerously. I have expressed my remorse to Andy and offered apologies about setting a bad example but he's always dismissed my feelings of responsibility.

Back to School

The summer following my brother's accident came to an end and I really hated having to return to school for my senior year. I felt I was abandoning my brother in his greatest time of need. When the morning I dreaded came, I went into Andy's room and cried as I watched him sleep.

That fall saw the Gulf Coast hit by multiple hurricanes including Hurricane Katrina which devastated New Orleans and due to the weather we had multiple days off from classes. My friends and I often joked, "My drinking problem was because I had two hands and only one mouth," and I used the school closings as an excuse to party. On one occasion the school's administration warned that any parties would result in campus security being deployed, but I had a little gathering anyway. That day the region was preparing for a category 5 hurricane with people filling the grocery stores to buy supplies. Fearing that I would be stuck in my apartment for days with the stores closed, I also headed to the grocery store to buy supplies; but for me that meant 3 cases of beer, ice, and rum from the neighboring liquor store. I was quite the spectacle in the store's checkout line. Women were coming up to me and saying, "You know honey, you really should buy some water and canned goods because this storm looks pretty bad." In my opinion, I already had all the essentials that I needed to ride out the storm in my carriage full of booze.

That night as the party and the weather got pretty crazy, the school announced that the campus was shutting down and every student should stay inside. Feeling quite a bit of liquid courage at this point of the evening, I asked a girl I knew for a thong, which turned out to be pink and see-through, and inspired by the movie "Old School" I changed into my "running gear", which meant just the thong, and tore off across campus in the midst of the storm. As I turned a blind corner, I ran directly into the headlights of a patrolling security vehicle and two officers jumped out and chased me. Under the influence and not thinking all that intelligently, I ran right into my apartment.

It wasn't long before the officers rapped on my door. I had not yet changed out of the "evidence" but I wasn't thinking so I answered the knocks still wearing the thong and nothing else. They filed a report and I was brought up on charges which required a meeting with the resident coordinator. Like I often did, I treated it like a joke and laughed about it with my drinking buddies. The resident coordinator asked me to defend my actions and give an example of how I contributed "anything positive to the university?"

I thought for a moment, stood up, looked her straight in the eye and said, "I have to be honest; I looked damn good in that thong."

Following my statement, I sat down and rested my case convinced I was going to be thrown out of school or at least the campus housing. The woman was quite amused with my brazen statement, and recommended no punishment beyond a note in my file. I just got very lucky to have someone with a sense of humor hearing my defense and once again, I got away with my bad behavior.

On another occasion, my drinking resulted in my doing something else unwise. My friends and I began to walk home after a night out at a bar across the Hillsborough River near campus. As we looked across the river at our building I decided it was "foolish" to walk all the way over the bridge when I could swim. Like a complete moron, I gave a friend my clothes to carry and dove in the filthy river and swam. Luckily one of my friends, a former competitive swimmer, dove in and accompanied me, because about halfway across the river I was spent and needed to be helped. My intoxication coupled with my poor swimming ability didn't help my chances. We made it across and immediately resumed partying in celebration. About twenty minutes later, the commotion of flashing lights and sirens brought us back to the river's edge. Apparently, a dead body had been floating down the river that night and the police were extracting the corpse only feet from where we had swam moments ago. Being quite drunk at the time I joked to my friends that "I knew I felt something in the water." But really, watching the police pull that body from the river made me realize how stupid and dangerous the swim had been. If only I had learned a lesson that night.

A College Graduate

My senior year went by in a blur. My brother's accident dominated my thoughts and frankly, I was drunk for most of the year. In retrospect, the drinking was an attempt to avoid the enormity of Andy's injury. By this time I had quit the golf team because it interfered with my social activities. I was a 23-year-old college senior content to take a test or two during the week and drink heavily Thursday from around 4 p.m. until about 3 a.m. Sunday morning. This routine lasted all year until graduation in May. My very supportive family made the trek south from the Boston area and the weekend was great. Despite seeing all of my loved ones, including my sister who came from California to celebrate during the weekend's festivities, I was depressed. Perhaps it was that now that I had finished college and reached what was supposed to be the start of my adult life, I still had no clue what I wanted to do, but that kind of worry is something many college grads must go through. I'm also an alcoholic, so the knowledge that the hard partying college lifestyle was ending got me down. Until that point I managed to maintain a fairly responsibility free life, and now I would be expected to be a self-supporting contributing member of society and stop my hard partying ways.

But that didn't happen. When I returned home my routine didn't change much, just the location of my incessant partying changed. I went to quite a few graduation parties and returned to my fun lifestyle. I went out to bars with friends almost every night, looking for a job in a lackadaisical way. Probably the best, and somewhat sober, weekend I had, was when I went up to Lake Winnipesaukee for motorcycle weekend with Kevin. Kevin's family, the Conway's, was always a great influence on me. His mom treats me like her son and I love her very much. If it wasn't for the respect I have for his mother, and the great support the Conway's showed me during my wilder years growing up, I probably would have done many other dangerous things in the years before my accident.

In one of my last clear memories from the months leading up to my accident, Kevin, his brother Marc, and I went on Marc's boat for a ride. When we got back from the ride, we came across a police standoff. An intoxicated motorcyclist had damaged multiple bikes on the boardwalk and was hiding in the cottage next door. After that weekend at Weirs Beach in early June, not much else of note happened until that one fateful night in July when my life changed completely.

"Jim, I can't go through this again."

The authorities couldn't get in touch with my family after I had been taken to Exeter Hospital on that early morning of July 4th, 2006. My license was old and had my previous residence listed, and we'd since moved to Maine. Only through good fortune did my parent's learn of my accident. A childhood girlfriend was in the room next to mine with her husband who had burned himself with fireworks. When she heard my name and that my family could not be located, she graciously shared that we had moved to Maine and the authorities were able to contact my parents at around 4 a.m.

My parents were startled awake by the late night phone call and my mom listened in shock as the voice on the line told her, "Your son has been in a car accident and is here at Exeter Hospital. By the time you get here, he'll be in transport to Beth Israel in Boston where they are better equipped to handle this type of situation, a serious head injury."

In shock, my mom hung up the phone and got out of bed.

"Is everything alright?" my father asked.

"No, you should get out of bed. We need to go to Boston right now. Jimmy's been in an accident," she said.

My father sprang into action telling one of my brother's friends, who had come to the house to celebrate the holiday, to feed Boomer, the family dog, and to lock up when he left. Then my father went upstairs to fill in the sleeping Andy. When my father came back downstairs, he found my mom rushing to pack a bag because she had no idea how long this trip would last.

As she packed, the tears streamed down her face. My mom looked at my dad and said, "Jim, I can't go through this again."

I feel horribly guilty for the pain my actions brought upon my family who only 14 months prior had dealt with my brother's accident. I can only imagine that the whole experience felt like one long terrible nightmare without reprieve. After taking care of the details about the dog and letting Andy know what had happened, my parents and brother began the hour-long trip to Boston full of fear and apprehension about what they would find.

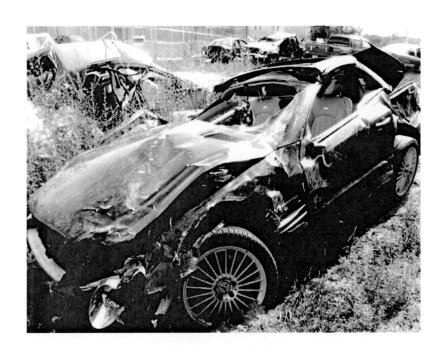

My Car after the crash on 7/4/06

**"Your son will wake up, but we don't
know what he'll be like."**

It was a very quiet ride to Boston for my family. As they
approached the city, my parents shared their fears with each other,
talking about what they would see. Hearing the words "serious head
injury" terrified my mom. They both expected to find me lying in a
bed with only bandages holding my head intact. They arrived to an
eerily quiet Boston despite the holiday.

After parking the car, the group headed to the ICU floor at
Beth Israel and tried to find the doctor in charge of my care. My
doctor, or any doctor for that matter, was nowhere to be found.
Thankfully, the nurses, Betsy and Vicki in particular, were
spectacular in keeping my family informed about what was going on
with me. My parents were told that I was being intubated—put on a
respirator to allow my brain to rest while the machine took breaths for
me. They would not be allowed to see me until the procedure was
finished. I was in a coma, and would remain so for over thirty hours,
so I couldn't share in my family's apprehension. After unsuccessfully
waiting around all day to see a doctor, they checked into a hotel after
finally seeing me.

Surprisingly, other than a few cuts and abrasions on my skin,
my mother describes me as looking peacefully at rest. Over the
course of the day they called Aimee, who was in San Diego for the
holiday, to fill her in. I hazily remember talking with Aimee on the

phone as she lay on a beach watching fireworks just before the accident on that fateful night. During our conversation I told her to dump her boyfriend because, "He didn't realize how lucky he was to have her." Aimee was in shock and immediately flew to Boston in her pajamas, once again traversing the country out of love for one of her brothers. The Clorox Company was incredibly understanding about the situation and my remarkable sister would stay and support the family for two months. Aimee's wonderful friend Kate, who lives in the Boston area, picked her up at the airport.

It would be two excruciating days before my parents saw a doctor. Although grateful to finally hear some news, the conversation wasn't pleasant. The doctor simply told my family I was stable and going to live.

My father implored, "Is he going to wake up?"

With my whole family awaiting his response, the doctor took a deep breath and said, "Your son will wake up, but we don't know what he will be like."

As happy as they were to know I would regain consciousness, this statement alarmed my family.

"Well, what does that mean?" my father asked.

The doctor told my family that I would regain consciousness, but he didn't know what consciousness would mean in terms of the level of function I would have. The doctor went on to explain that the cat scans showed that I had sustained a severe traumatic brain injury (TBI). I had experienced a diffuse axonal injury, a closed head injury in which momentum causes the axons, which connect the brain's cells to each other, to separate. Brain axons are literally sheared and the damage cannot be fully assessed in the acute or early stage. The injury is particularly damaging because it affects many of the brain's functions indiscriminately and only ten percent of individuals who lose consciousness ever regain awareness. The only way I can even fathom the emotions my family felt is in remembering the absolute denial of reality I felt, and still do sometimes, surrounding Andy's injury.

He's Awake

I woke up on July 6th, two days after my accident, but "awake" didn't quite mean what my family expected. Their fairy tale was to come into my room to find me smiling and talking, but that was not to be. In my case, "awake" meant I had simply opened my eyes. I don't remember anything from this period of my hospitalization, but I'm told my family was amazing. Grampy, the paternal grandfather I first visited Tampa with, had suffered a stroke only a couple of years earlier and no longer drove, or was supposed to, but he drove in to see me almost every day. Jim Scott the first, or just "Senior" as many workers at the pet food business called him, has played many roles in my life. Because I went to college close to where he lives half the year, I have been fortunate to spend a lot of time with him. In relaxed moments he provides comic relief to almost any situation. In any teaching moment that presents itself, a relevant story from years in business is told. My relationship with Grampy has become even stronger over time, with all that has happened, growing into an incredible friendship.

My cousin Mike, one of my best friends, came in every night and watched Red Sox games with me and Betsy, my incredible nurse. Mike was in so much that he became close with all the nurses. In fact, after a game got over late he would often sleep in my room. My mom could never understand how Mike got a cot, yet when she stayed in my room she slept on a chair. I appreciate these visits so much because I imagine that I wasn't great company. I couldn't even speak yet. I give Mike a hard time for being my elder (one year my senior) so escaping all of my jokes was probably a relief for him. We banter back and forth all the time.

Once Mike commented on my speech returning and said, "Jim, do you remember when you couldn't talk for 5 weeks?"

I didn't recall and was silent. Mike went on, "That was great." That's still hysterical to me, only because Mike said it and it's probably true.

Mike's brother Matt also came in to visit when he heard that I was "awake." As my Nana recounts, he was also devastated to find that "awake" meant that I had merely opened my eyes. To everyone, the vision of "awake" meant I was back to my pre-injury self, not that I was in a vegetative state. When Matt came out of my room Nana remembers the horribly terrified look on his face.

"What are they talking about? Jim's not awake," he exclaimed.

Finally, on July 10, I became medically stable. I wasn't going to die. Now "out of the woods," the doctors switched my breathing functions from a respirator to a tracheotomy tube, which allowed me to perform a greater percentage of breathing on my own, a positive step. They also inserted a feeding tube, another stride forward. I was taken off sedation and became a little more alert. The feeding tube was very important because I had lost so much weight—nearly 10 lbs in just a week—and I could finally receive some much needed nourishment. I would ultimately drop 30 pounds during my 3 months of hospitalization.

As I continued to make strides my family thought about the next steps. It was obvious that due to the severity of my injuries, I would need acute inpatient rehabilitation. They had experienced firsthand the wonderful rehabilitation services my brother received at Spaulding Rehabilitation Hospital and my family chose it as the next step in my recovery as well. On August 3rd I was transferred to Spaulding, a place all too familiar to the Scott family.

A small step in the right direction

My family was very excited to see me begin the rehabilitation phase of my recovery. As I got used to my new surroundings, Dr. Heechin Chae, the director of the brain injury floor at Spaulding, introduced himself to my family as the doctor in charge of my case, a far cry from the tortuous wait my parents had experienced at BI, my family was very appreciative. Dr. Chae is a wonderful man, a very compassionate person, and a great doctor. He took the time to explain things in terms that my parents could understand as well as laying out a plan for my care. A team of therapists was put in place in order to achieve the best outcome for me. For Physical Therapy (PT), I worked with Steve and Wendy. Steve is an incredibly knowledgeable therapist and I loved working with him because he had a way of pushing me to work hard that motivated me. Wendy was awesome. She has a great sense of humor and took on a very compassionate and supportive role in working with me. For Occupational Therapy (OT) I was assigned Morgan, who I really liked working with and not just because she's so cute. She's a very skilled therapist with a great attitude and she always encouraged me to work hard. By then I had just started speaking and was set up to work with Julia, a speech therapist. As I gained alertness, speech therapy became quite enjoyable. My thinking seemed fairly clear, although I told Julia that the accident was 3 days ago when in reality it had been over a month and a half.

How I began to speak again is a funny story that brought much needed humor into the grim circumstances. While I was still at BI, my mom was visiting me by herself. As I was lying in my bed, I looked at her somewhat annoyed prompting her to ask, "What's wrong?" Without skipping a beat I responded as if nothing was odd about my suddenly speaking. "Mom, its f***ing hot in here," I complained. Although not thrilled by my language she was excited that I had finally spoken and immediately called my Aunt Diane to tell her the news. Aunt Diane, who is also my Godmother and has always spoiled me, immediately drove in to visit with a fan. She's a phenomenal, caring lady. She'd give us all ginger ale to help with a stomach ache as kids or stay with either me or Andy when our parents had to travel after our accidents.

That same day my mom had my brother on the phone and I said, "What's up?" to him. This really pumped my brother up because he was very distraught about my accident. On that same day my friend Larry came in and excited to hear that I was talking, he tried to converse with me. He grabbed my bicep and commented, "Look at this, my arms are bigger than yours now." After thinking of a smart ass comment, I replied "You're jealous." It was the typical ribbing banter that we often exchanged and it gave Larry and my mom great hope because it was a glimpse of the pre-injury Jim's personality they hadn't seen for a while. In one more "old Jim" moment I quoted a movie line that my brother and I love. Ashley, Larry's then girlfriend and now wife, commented that, "I can't wait to hear him say 'Oh herrro'." Upon hearing this I said the phrase from the movie "Team America: World Police", cracking up the room.

Once at Spaulding, I did well in my new rehab routine and was making good progress when I suddenly became sick. The incision from where my feeding tube was inserted had created scar tissue that blocked my small intestine with food building up because it couldn't be digested. The details are disgusting so I won't go into them, but I was extremely ill and kept vomiting. On August 10, just a week after I left, I was back in a hospital bed at Beth Israel.

My family was pretty upset with this seemingly huge setback. I had to go back to where I had been when I was in a coma, despite that I was doing so well at Spaulding. The blockage was working itself out and the doctor and my family were eager for me to return to Spaulding. After a week of rest and a lot of vomiting, I was scheduled to return to Spaulding a week later, on August 18. Up until that date I remember nothing about my life since the accident and until this point in the story, I've relied entirely on the meticulous notes taken by my Mother to recall what happened. My first memory of my post accident life began on August 18, six weeks after the accident, and the ambulance ride back to Spaulding. This probably has a lot to do with regaining my ability to talk, as I believe people always remember things better when they actively participate in them. Perhaps high school would have gone a little smoother had I realized this back then, but you live, you learn—at least that's how they say it's supposed to go. The rest of my story is a much more Jim-centric version of events.

I returned to the very familiar Spaulding to stay for a while and jumped back into the routine of PT and OT in the morning, followed by Speech in the afternoon. Around this time my speech therapist, Julia, informed me that she would be moving to L.A. with her boyfriend who was enrolling at USC. I was sad because she was great and I enjoyed working with her. In one of our last sessions, she wanted me to work on increasing the volume of my voice and asked me to make a list of words I routinely spoke loudly to practice with. We had a good laugh when I asked, "Should this list be rated PG?" The only words I could think of were all of the four letter variety.

My sadness miraculously subsided when I met Julia's replacement, Katie. Katie was one of the most attractive women I had ever seen and I thrilled to begin working with her. I suddenly got alot more concerned with my appearance and often requested extra showers and shaves. The nursing staff at Spaulding was incredible. Three nurses in particular, Corrine, Richard, and Janice were tremendous.

Corrine could not have been nicer to me and my family. Whenever she was working, she asked me who my visitors would be that day and when the list included a female she said, "Well we need to shave then. I want my boy looking good." When she finished, she rubbed my face to check the job. She just wanted to make sure I felt like a human being and make my time in the hospital comfortable, which I appreciate more than she'll ever know.

Richard is an awesome guy. He's meticulous in his appearance, always wears a tie, and takes the same pride in his work. My scalp was quite dry from lying on a pillow all day so Aunt Diane brought me in some T-gel. Richard would follow the directions to a "T", looking at his watch and timing how long he left the shampoo on my hair before rinsing, a daily routine which showed how much pride he took in his work, and that he truly cared about us patients. It was great talking about sports and other "guy" stuff with Richard.

Janice was the night shift (3-11p.m.) nurse and on duty when Mike and I watched many of the Red Sox games. Although the Sox had a tough end to their season, having Mike and Janice there made my time in the hospital bearable. A typical guy, I nearly had a nervous breakdown whenever I couldn't find my TV remote and would call Janice in to help, which she always did. She never complained. Her great attitude and smile that could light up a room were a great comfort during that tough time for me.

Homeward bound

As the summer ended and fall began, I was desperate to go home. A meeting was scheduled to discuss my discharge plan. My dad had to take the day off to attend and I remember joking about the times my misbehavior in school required him to appear at meetings about me. He laughed, saying, "Yeah, but this is a meeting I'm excited about." My parents came in early to visit me.

My mom asked, "Is there anything you want me to say on your behalf, Jim?"

I replied, "Just get me the f*** out of here."

The typical inpatient Jim was back which made my mom ever more certain I was ready to leave the hospital. Because many patients suffering a TBI require nursing home-care upon discharge, my living situation at home was discussed. The Spaulding staff was relieved to hear that my house had a shower chair and even an elevator, and was prepared for my arrival. I can only imagine how difficult the transition could have been had my parents not already equipped the house for my brother.

After the meeting, a date of Tuesday, October 3 was set as my discharge date and I was excited to have a light at the end of the tunnel. I'd been itchy to go home and kept asking for an earlier discharge but my mom would say, "We want you to walk out of this hospital." I knew she was right and hoped to be physically "fixed" by the time of my discharge, a hope that proved to be unrealistic. I left the hospital in a wheelchair although I was able to walk with a cane. When he heard of my discharge, my Uncle Tom came right in to Boston to help my mom and I pack up. This was incredibly nice of him, but it was also necessary because he had to lift me into my mother's truck.

As it turned out I actually got discharged six days early. On Wednesday, September 27th as my mom headed in to see me that morning her cell phone rang. "Hi Janet, this is John (my case manager) from Spaulding. I just got off the phone with Blue Cross and they want Jimmy out on Friday, not next Tuesday. Will that be ok for your family?"

My mom had already prepared the house and replied that it was. After hanging up, my mom thought about how nice it would be not to make the long drive to Boston from Maine each day because she'd just have to go upstairs to see me instead. A moment later the phone rang again. "It's John again. They actually want him out today." My mom frantically called my father, who was in a meeting, and his secretary passed him a note with the news. When my mom finally arrived, I was in PT with Wendy and Steve. She told them the news and a bit shocked, Steve said, "Well we need to get him ready with some stairs then."

The four of us —Wendy, Steve, my mom, and I—headed to a huge staircase behind the hospital. To me, the ascent looked like Mt. Everest and Wendy was a bit worried about my being able to climb the stairs.

"Steve, are you sure about this?" she asked.

"Well, if he's headed home today, he needs to be ready," Steve replied and I was off.

My mom watched nervously as I slowly made progress up the stairs. When I finally reached the top, Steve and I exchanged high fives. I felt like Sir Edmund Hilary as I looked down those stairs. Steve was absolutely correct that all that therapy activity would prepare me for discharge. After completing the climb, I was confident in my ability to navigate the not always accessible world.

Plans were made to pick up my AFO, an assistive walking brace, on the way home, and after my Uncle Tom hoisted me into the truck, we were off. I was pumped as we got on Rt.1 via the Tobin Bridge. The ride was filled with excitement, as I could not wait to get home and hang out with my dog Boomer. Mentally, I was in complete denial about my injury and thought I'd be back to "normal" in a few months.

My mom showed incredible foresight in handling my discharge. She didn't want me to fall out of the rehab routine that Spaulding had created and set things in motion for me to begin rehab in Kennebunk, ME, at River Ridge. Since I was discharged six days early things also had to be accelerated at home. As she always does, my mom found a way to get the best for me, and I started rehab right away.

Same Story, Different Setting

River Ridge, an inpatient/outpatient rehabilitation facility about 30 minutes from my home, is a great neurological rehab center. I was thrilled to be waking up in my own house and commuting to rehab instead of living in a hospital.

I quickly became acclimated to River Ridge and its great staff of therapists. I had Tina for PT. Tina is young and I felt I could really relate to her. My OT therapist was Melanie assisted by a student intern Debbie. They were also young and had great attitudes that provided me with constant support. At River Ridge, I also had speech therapy with Ellen, a great person for me to work with because she had a good sense for my needs. My actual speech was fairly good by this time so we focused more on my executive skills. This involved some homework and for the first time in my life I was a good pupil, completing all the assignments. I actually enjoyed the work because it broke up my boring days after leaving rehab. My progression from wheelchair to walking on my own is a good example of my stubbornness and impatience actually serving me well. I was in a wheelchair when I began at River Ridge. Gradually, as my walking improved at rehab, I left the wheelchair in my mom's truck despite the suggestions of Tina. Finally, we compromised and decided I would use a cane when walking. As time went on I would often "forget" to bring the cane to rehab. Eventually, I was cane free.

Boomer

While there are certainly many reasons that I have progressed as well as I have, my "little yellow friend," as I liked to call Boomer, played a huge role. My father often speaks of the "power of pets" on their owners when he speaks from a marketing standpoint in his capacity as a pet food company employee. This whole experience has made me a believer. My dog, Boomer, a yellow lab, has since passed away, but he was, as my often says, truly bionic. As a puppy, he blew out ligaments in every leg and had many surgeries. As he got older, Boomer had cancer and underwent chemotherapy. As a food crazy yellow lab, he suffered no loss of appetite from chemo. On one occasion he jumped up and cleaned out the candy dish on the counter in the vet's waiting room after just completing a chemo session.

As a typical lazy kid, I never wanted to take Boomer out for walks but that changed when I first came home from the hospital. I set a goal to walk Boomer alone and worked hard to reach it. In the beginning, Boomer actually walked me. I still had a cane, and with limited use of my left arm, I couldn't hold both the leash and my cane at the same time. My dad, Boomer and I would take walks which were essentially therapy for me. Eventually, I no longer used a cane and began taking him myself. At first I only walked in our yard so my parents could make sure I didn't fall. After a while, I circled the entire neighborhood. It was going great and I really improved my walking. Mondays, however, were a difficult day for my walks with

Boomer because it was trash day in my parent's neighborhood and Boomer liked to rip apart trash bags looking for scraps. At about 75 lbs and strong, he easily overpowered me on trash day. He'd smell some particularly enticing trash and pull the leash so hard that I'd go flying and tumble to the ground. I left Mondays to my parents but in the winter when it was around zero degrees and snowing outside—just plain nasty—I'd feed Boomer and trudge through the snow, every day but Monday, with him for about a mile while he took his time going to the bathroom. I truly believe Boomer played a huge role in my progress and honestly think Blue Cross should've sent him a check.

For a period of time when I was living alone in Portsmouth, Boomer was my only companion. I typically become increasingly depressed as the days get shorter and the temperature drops. When Boomer ran the show, which was the entire time we lived together, he provided me with a responsibility. Every morning he'd wake me up around 6:00 a.m. with a nudge in the chest courtesy of his nose. I'd enthusiastically get out of bed, amazing from a kid who was tardy for school over 50% of the time, and precisely measure a cup of dry food mixed with a tablespoon of wet, canned food. Of course, the food had to be mixed with warm water. I cherished this responsibility as it provided distraction from my dark thoughts. Boomer became a celebrity in Portsmouth and people always asked about him. They still do which brings me back to those days as his "father".

Boomer could be an absolute misfit when any food was within 500 yards, but was the sweetest dog with people. Children approached him and put their fingers into his mouth and ears while pulling his tail with the other hand. I loved that dog and he still lives in my fond memories. One snowy night he awoke me around 4:00 a.m. with his whimpering, so uncommon I immediately got up and pulled on some winter gear. We made our way out to the windy streets and he took his time looking for the perfect spot. Having finished the job, we headed home and I slipped on some ice, falling on by back. I held Boomer's leash with my good hand while unsuccessfully trying to stand. Finally, I let go of this leash, petrified that he would wander off, but he just stood there staring at me. I kept saying, "Stay here, Boom, stay here." Wouldn't you know it, he actually stayed. By the look on his face it was obvious he was quite perturbed that my fall had interrupted his walk. I kept struggling and as I resigned myself to failure, a long haul trucker who had pulled over for the night saw me on the sidewalk, got out of his truck, and helped me up. My heart was racing as we walked home where I lay down on Boomer's pillow with him and laughed at myself.

Even More Rehab

In the late fall, I went back in to Spaulding to see Dr. Chae for a routine checkup. He asked how things were going and I expressed my frustration at my seemingly slow progress. He told me to be patient and recognize the great strides I had made, but that one avenue I could explore was aquatic therapy. My mom and I were excited that there was something else that could help my recovery. We quickly decided that my mom would look for the nearest aquatic therapy pool so we could supplement the wonderful services I was receiving at River Ridge. After making a few exploratory phone calls, my mother found Portsmouth Regional Hospital Rehab located conveniently nearby and we made an appointment for an afternoon following my rehab at River Ridge. It was then that I first met Barb, a very nice and tremendously knowledgeable physical therapist. I really enjoyed the pool and was amazed by all the equipment at the facility. To me it was just another gym, like the ones I had worked out at for years. The services at River Ridge were great, but I thought I would thrive in a more aggressive program and we all decided that I would switch to Portsmouth full time. I started Day Rehab, an intensive program beginning at 8:00 a.m. until lunchtime Monday and Wednesday. On Tuesday and Thursday, I ate lunch at the facility before going in the pool from 1-2:00 p.m. I was very excited to make the switch.

I met my rehab team that first day and quickly learned that one great thing about Portsmouth Rehab is how much all the therapists work together, a team approach that works very well. For PT, I worked with Barb whose enthusiasm brought out my best effort. OT was handled by Mary, a wonderful mother of five who I had a lot of fun with. By then my speech therapy had shifted focus to more advanced cognitive skills and memory with Carolyn put in charge of that. She was always honest with me and allowed me to pick my own areas to work on. Dr. Joan Breen ran the facility and treated me like a son. Rounding out the team was Jeremiah, a rehab aid around my age. He's a great kid and we became good friends. He made me look forward to rehab every day because it was like going to the gym with a buddy. The schedule was great because I was the only one in the pool during my sessions with Jeremiah so as I worked hard, Jeremiah and I would crack ourselves up quoting funny movies and trading humorous stories.

Another benefit of Day Rehab at Portsmouth was that I really enjoyed my interactions with the other clients. Golf was a passion for many at Day Rehab and I talked golf with a great guy named Charlie. After he learned I was a golfer in college and wanted to play again, I was set up to work with an awesome guy named Frank whose passion was golf. About once a week I had one of my PT sessions with Frank working on my golf game. I really enjoyed these sessions and credit them with reintroducing me to the game.

I also met a really nice man named Steve, who only lived about two miles from our house in Cape Neddick. A stroke had left him in a wheelchair and without the ability to talk but through his hard work and perseverance, Steve is now talking and gets around on his own two feet. I also met a very intelligent college student, Tessa, who had also been in a car accident. Tessa returned to and graduated from Brandeis University after her TBI, which is something I greatly admire because I now know the effects of a brain injury and went back to school myself. It's incredibly difficult to be in an educational environment after a severe head injury.

Rehab was going well and I was able to walk without a brace or a cane. I eagerly anticipated playing some golf as the summer approached.   I began by playing a few shots here and there, progressing to the point that I could walk some and play 18 holes. It was my goal to walk 18 holes and I was determined to do it. For my 25th birthday my parents took me up to Samoset Resort in Camden, Maine, a place I love. I started the round walking and although exhausted, I was determined to finish that way.   By the 16th hole I could barely stand up. My mom pleaded with me to get in the cart but I stubbornly refused and finished the round. I was a scratch golfer in college (shooting around par, which is 72 at Samoset), but was happy finishing all 18 holes that day. I added up the score and laughed because my score of 140—68 on the front and 72 on the back—had 9-hole scores that equaled some of my past scores for all 18 holes. My diminished skills on the golf course are a good example of the adjustments I've had to, and continue to, make due to my diminished physical abilities. Now that I've lived in this "new" body for six years, I think I've accepted my altered abilities fairly well and the dissonance between my expectations and reality has closed, but not entirely.

The World of Work

I did play a lot of golf that summer, but I had some responsibilities as well. I was a college graduate and both my parents and I thought I should begin my career. Ideally, I would use my economics degree by working in the financial services field, which I am interested in. Prior to my accident I had met with Lisa, my grandparents' financial advisor at Smith Barney and brainstormed some ideas for my future. I have always been fond of Lisa because she is incredibly nice and very intelligent; and she's originally from Maine, which gives us something in common. While in Tampa, I drove to Naples to celebrate Grampy's 80th birthday, which Lisa and her parents also attended. I really liked her parents and had a great time, so I was excited when I found out that Lisa would be willing to have me intern in her Boston office.

The people at Smith Barney were incredibly nice and I gained much from the experience. Lisa handled me with unbelievable compassion for my injury while making me feel valuable at the same time. My main responsibilities were to maintain a database of business leaders and research the investment products that Lisa requested me to look into. One great thing was the access to Citigroup Investment Research's research tools. While the technical and research experience I gained was great, I also made tremendous strides from a recovery standpoint at the internship.

The commute to Boston's Post Office Square from Maine, although long and tiring, was very beneficial. I had to take the train from Exeter, NH which made me follow the train schedule and develop time management skills. I also had to interact with the general public on the train and as I talked with fellow commuters, I slowly gained confidence in my speaking ability, confidence which had been sorely lacking. I began to see that I could be a contributing member of society.

I interned at Smith Barney through the summer and early fall and while I loved the people, the commute was draining. At the end of the fall, Genie Wallace, the mom of a former elementary school classmate, offered to introduce me to her financial planner in the hope that he could offer me some help in finding work closer to home. I met Charlie Peckham, Mrs. Wallace's financial planner, who was extremely nice and said he would think about it and let me know some ideas.

A few days later, a wonderful woman named Marilyn Morrison called and asked me to come into Charlie's Exeter, NH office and meet her to discuss an idea. Marilyn was Charlie's SEC licensed assistant and office manager and she offered me a job as a research assistant at his company in the Commonwealth Financial Network. I was thrilled and started at two days a week while continuing rehab, but while I was making great physical progress, I wasn't faring well mentally. Sadly, I had to leave because my depression became unmanageable.

Into the Darkness

I vividly remember the first time I thought of suicide. It was during April vacation of my 7th grade year and the whole family was on vacation in Italy. We were in Rome, staying in two hotel rooms on the fifth or sixth floor. The family was excited to get out and see the city and stood in the hallway eager to leave. As they knocked on the door to get my attention, I stood by the window with its wide open shutters. There was no glass or screen to stop me as I looked down to the piazza below wondering if the fall would kill me. The thought of returning to school and what I saw as a pointless life tormented me. I tried to will myself to jump.

Looking back, I realize I've been depressed since long before my accident. I was an active alcoholic from age 16 on and often thought I would rather be dead than fail at living up to the impossible expectations I set for myself. When I was young, these unrealistic expectations and goals were to play in the NHL or on the PGA tour, but as I grew up, they became what I thought were quite reasonable— I would graduate college and be a rich hotshot businessman. Maybe I suddenly realized this goal was unrealistic and that I would never have the kind of life that I had imagined and I had a death wish. I wasn't actively trying to kill myself through the typical manners of suicide, but I was living my life very recklessly. I partied all the time without giving thought to my safety or well being, with ultimately my alcohol use and recklessness leading to my accident.

The drinking in that hotel room on the weekend of that hockey tournament when I was a teen was merely a precursor of the problem that would plague me for almost 10 years until my accident. My parents warned me about alcohol. They both have strong histories of alcoholism in their families and often mentioned that alcoholism was heavily genetic and that I needed to be careful. I love and respect my parents tremendously and know they love all of their children very much. There's no question about that, but while my parents showed great fear and understanding of the genetic predisposition faced by their children towards alcoholism, our home was always completely stocked with alcohol.

After that first drink, I was a practicing alcoholic by the time I reached my sophomore year of high school. The problem of getting booze was a non-issue for me because I often stole it from my parents. Although Andy is much younger than I am, our drinking overlapped when I was home from college on breaks. Shamefully enough, at the peak of our partying Andy and I were probably stealing a gallon of liquor a week as well as a good number of beers from the garage. One thing that I take from this knowledge is that, understanding the genetic factors of alcoholism, the parents of kids with a genetic predisposition towards alcoholism should rid their homes of any easily accessed alcohol. I am terrified to have any children because I know I will pass this tendency on to them, but if I do the house will be dry other than what guests bring or my wife personally drinks.

There's a balance between understanding that alcohol played a part in both of our accidents and recognizing that I am an adult who made a horrible decision and must take responsibility. My need to take responsibility and my incredible guilt has caused me deep psychological problems since my accident, including a deep depression and self-loathing so intense that I am at times suicidal. On four occasions I've been hospitalized for mental health treatment, once following a suicide attempt in which I tried to cut my wrists, once after an overdose on, ironically, antidepressants. On the other two occasions, I asked for help before I could make another attempt.

There are still times when I ponder suicide and it terrifies me because I don't truly want to die. I recognize the possibility that my life will have a worthwhile future. The frightening truth is that at times, if I had access to a gun my life would be over. A great friend and mentor of mine named Barry Dyke often reminds me that suicide is a permanent solution to temporary problems. Recently I heard a speaker reinforce this belief when he told of his son coming home from school.

When the boy came in the house his father asked, "How was your day?" The son's response was beautifully simple, yet accurate.

"It was a good day," he said, "with a few bad moments."

The young boy makes the profound statement that I'm still realizing —ride out the bad spots and the totality is pretty good.

I've maintained continuous sobriety since my accident on July 4. 2006 so I've overcome addiction, right? Not really. My addiction, which I choose to call alcoholism, now manifests itself in obsessive-compulsive behaviors. In my youth, it was the socially acceptable pursuit of athletic achievement, then alcohol took over. Addictions come in many varieties and serve an important function. For me, and countless others, my addictive thoughts and behaviors serve as a way to handle emotions. I have trouble dealing with the ever-changing feelings that all humans experience. This was true before my accident and has only become more difficult due to the significant damage to the frontal lobe of my brain, the area of the brain that regulates emotion. Coincidentally, most of the damage to my brain occurred in the frontal lobe as the momentum of the car slammed my brain into the front of my skull causing a large bleed as well as the shearing of axons or nerve fibers.

Swapping Addictions

I was suddenly sober. My accident was awful but I'm incredibly lucky that no one else was hurt and I got the gift of instantaneous sobriety. Without my usual anesthetic I find it intolerable to process my emotions, good or bad and immediately a food and weight obsession filled the void drinking left. When I entered the hospital after my accident I weighed 165 pounds. When I left Spaulding, I was 135 pounds. I was consumed by anxiety about gaining weight, obsessed with staying below 140 pounds. Hey, what better way of self-punishment and keeping my thoughts predictable than starving myself, right? I kept a running tab of my daily calorie intake in my head, getting a sense of accomplishment and success by keeping my eating to a minimum. I began to gain weight when I started eating real food in the hospital, and was terrified that I would never stop gaining. In outpatient rehab I was weighed weekly for the purpose of completing progress notes to send to the insurance company and when I saw the number increase, even slightly, I felt threatened by the change. I was hyper-focused on the numerical measurements of my progress and felt my weight was a number that I could control even if I'd lost control over some physical movements. I took pride in keeping the number below a benchmark I chose, that I had control over. The mental exhaustion and anxiety this pattern of eating caused left no room for reflection on how I'd really thrown a wrench in my life plan, all of which was the purpose of this obsession to begin with.

As I returned to an extremely low weight and my eating practices grew more restrictive, the people around me noticed and suggested I get help for my eating issue. During the winter of '07 I began a day treatment program running from 7 a.m.-7 p.m. I was living in Southern Maine and I received treatment in Portland. My thinking was still quite foggy and I resisted change so I didn't gain much from the experience. I did, however, begin eating a more appropriate, although still restrictive diet.

Flash forward to two years later, the day after Christmas in '09. I was admitted to an inpatient treatment hospital in Wisconsin. Again, I resisted help and discharged myself from the 30 day program after only six days. Then, in June of 2012, with my 30th birthday approaching, I flew to St. Louis to a residential treatment center specializing in trauma and eating disorders. I thought I would be there for four weeks, but ended up staying for six. I had my six year anniversary of my accident, the day marking six years of sobriety, and my 30th birthday at the treatment center. Overall, the experience was good as I learned a lot about myself and the underlying issues I face.

Unfortunately, my motivation for recovery ebbs and flows. At times my anxiety builds to a point where I feel that I'm about to spontaneously combust. My thoughts race at moments like these and I seem to act in absurd ways, whether by binge eating, dropping classes from my course schedule or out of school completely. I cancel plans for activities I know will be enjoyable, getting instant relief or a calm feeling from completely retreating from the world and any uncertainty life might present. The key for my psychological health and living the most productive life possible will be learning to tolerate this anxiety without acting compulsively.

After my accident my parents told me I had fallen asleep while driving. They were trying to protect me but when discovering I faced felony DWI charges it forced them to tell me the truth in August of 2007. I faced jail time and heavy fines in addition to the obvious license suspension. I was shocked and deeply troubled. I sweated out my future for a few months and only when a Strafford

County, NH Assistant DA showed me great compassion was I offered a plea deal. I plead guilty, lost my license for 2 years (3 and a half total), and paid $1600 in fines.

That part of the ordeal was over but incessant worrying and anxiety about my fate coupled with my Post Traumatic Stress Disorder (PTSD) triggered a depression so deep that it ultimately led to my being hospitalized numerous times. At first it was just the legal issue, but as I began to face the permanency of my disability the depression worsened. As I began to make seemingly positive strides, these accomplishments only forced me to face the reality of my disability.

It would hit me in many ways, at any time. My mom had to dress me for work each morning because the limited use of my left arm inhibits my ability to put on business attire. It was particularly difficult, even impossible, for me to button my pants and I lived in constant fear that I'd have to use the bathroom and lower my pants.

One day, my fear came true. I was stuck in a stall with my pants down for about 20 minutes. I couldn't yell for help because the restroom at my work was in the hall of a large office complex. Finally, a total stranger came in, used the urinal, and went to the sink to wash his hands. I swallowed my pride and asked him for help. To exit the stall, I had to use the hand holding up my pants in order to turn the latch. My pants fell to my ankles as I let go of them. Suddenly, the man saw me standing with my pants around my ankles in the mirror's reflection. A look of shock crossed his face as I said, "Sir, I assure you I'm not a weirdo, but do you think you could help me pull my pants up and tuck in my shirt?" After I explained my situation, the man was incredibly nice and helped me out. He was incredibly compassionate and said, "In the future, I don't want you stuck in here, so here's my business card. I work in this building and want you to bring your cell phone with you, and call me if you ever need help again." I carried that wonderful man's card the whole time I worked there, just in case.

I still face many physical difficulties and am also mourning the death of the old me. I can no longer do many of the things I once did, and as time passes, I realize I'll probably never be able to do them again. I feel guilty all the time because I know my current condition is entirely my fault. I simply cannot forgive myself, and although I know I need to, I doubt I ever will completely. I only managed my depression through medication and the help of Psychiatrists, first Dr. Ilene Spitzer of Portsmouth, and then Dr. George Hilton in Dover. I had a wonderful relationship with Dr. Spitzer. I felt like she really "got" me and that I could tell her anything. Because of my disability, I feel like people are overly nice to me. Dr. Spitzer, on the other hand wasn't afraid to highlight my faulty thinking and irrational thoughts, which I appreciated. It was refreshing to have honest conversations with someone who had my best interest in mind. Dr. Hilton was a great fit for me because he is very knowledgeable about brain injury having worked at an inpatient facility specializing in brain injury. Unfortunately, Dr. Hilton retired so now I work with Dr. Mendoza in Portsmouth.

I've worked with four psychotherapists since my accident. Each therapist has provided extensive talk therapy and a great outlet for me to voice my frustrations. First I worked with Candace Wheeler, whose office is within 200 yards from my condo in Portsmouth. The close proximity of her office came in handy as I had lost my license for such a lengthy period of time.

As I developed an eating disorder and it worsened, I sought help from a social worker, Pat Meyers, specializing in the field. I attended a support group in her office with other individuals struggling with eating disorders. The group provided a comfortable place to discuss my struggles and helped me realize I wasn't the only person suffering from an eating disorder. I was advised to begin dialectical behavior therapy (DBT) and began working with Beth-Salve Hudgins on modifying my thoughts.

I gave up hope and felt pretty helpless about my struggle and stopped receiving therapy altogether but my experiment of living without any therapy whatsoever was miserable. It got to the point that I rarely left my place, living in isolation. A friend recommended a therapist who had authored a book on Anorexia and I contacted her: Monika Ostroff of Exeter, NH, just a 20 minute drive from me, and after my consult with her, I knew it was a great match. I'm quite sarcastic and tend to speak in analogies making abstract connections to prove my point. This doesn't work with Monika and she calls me on my bulls**t quite often. I've been working with Monika for over two years and make as much progress as I'm willing to, but that willingness varies with the fluctuations in my stubbornness. At this point Monika is completely on to me and many of my extremely faulty thinking patterns, which is a good thing, I guess.

The Krempels Center

It was due to my depression and subsequent hospitalization that I left my job in November of '08. The newfound time I had on my hands provided the perfect opportunity for me to explore a program I had heard about at Portsmouth Rehab. The program at The Krempels Center—then called Stepping Stones—is in Portsmouth at the beautiful Community Campus. It's a 3 day a week program for people living with acquired brain injury and runs from 9:40 am until 1:50 pm with a choice of morning and afternoon groups in addition to a community meeting each morning. The wonderful thing about The Krempels Center is the terrific staff and that it offers all brain injury survivors a place to feel welcomed.

My time at The Krempels Center has been incredible. I usually arrive at 9:40 to hang out and play cards, or talk sports with Hank, a great guy who knows everything about baseball. It's a nice way to start the day, then it's off to community meeting where daily announcements are made and member news is shared. Following the meeting I usually participate in some sort of support group which provides an opportunity to talk about things all of us members with brain injuries can relate to. The morning groups run from 11 a.m. until lunchtime at noon and after lunch I often play mentally challenging and fun games in Brain Power. This offers me the chance to challenge myself in a non-judgmental environment and is very fun although I'm frequently overmatched by some of the other members.

Jim Scott

I've met many admirable people at The Krempels Center. Not only are the staff members incredibly nice and supportive, but all of the members of the community are great friends. Two in particular have perhaps the most incredible smiles I have ever seen—Jacki Mike and Phyllis Burkl. I love the whole program, but I would go just to see their smiles. With Jacki, it is usually good news about the Red Sox that brings a smile to her face, but with Phyllis, I just seem to amuse her. I hope it's not my looks.

Another great benefit of the program is the interaction with all the interns. Not only are they vital to the center's success, but they also have wonderfully compassionate and caring personalities that are displayed on a daily basis through the great work that they do.

Again?

Prior to becoming a member at KC, I did have another visit to the hospital, only this time; it was a step in the right direction. In November of '07 I underwent Achilles lengthening surgery to deal with an ankle contracture that resulted from my months of hospitalization. Because I was off my feet for so long my Achilles tendon shortened which limited my ability to raise and clear the toes of my left foot when walking. I had countless Botox shots to try to loosen the tendon and worked tirelessly with Jeremiah at Portsmouth Day Rehab to stretch my ankle with the slant board and also with the ultrasound machine.

The surgery itself went well. I woke up in the recovery room and a nurse asked me questions to see if I was mentally alert. Questions like, "Do you know what day it is?" and "Who is the President?" which have become all too familiar after my months of hospitalization. After those typical questions she asked me if I was ok and was a bit puzzled when I pointed at my father and said, "You should be asking him if he's alright." When she asked what I meant, I said that he had just had surgery as well. "Oh my really, on what?" she asked. "Well it was a fairly invasive procedure where they removed his head from his ass," I replied. My family immediately knew I was feeling all right.

After the surgery, I was in a cast with my ankle in a neutral position for a month in order to allow the tendon time to heal. When the cast was removed my leg brace was locked in the neutral position (a right angle) to keep stress off the tendon. The outcome of the surgery was good and I returned to rehab. I looked forward to working on my recovery again with the great team of therapists at Portsmouth Rehab and having some laughs with Jeremiah in our pool group. I also continued OT to work on the function of my left arm, which was, and still is, slowly improving.

Insurance

It's important to point out that insurance is a very important issue for people with TBI's and for everyone. I had Blue Cross at the time of my accident and they were very generous in extending my coverage despite the fact that I was no longer a student and as such not covered under my father's plan. The troubling thing is that I was only allowed 100 rehab sessions that first year, which is considered extraordinary coverage. This sounds like a lot, but with 12 visits per week, the allotment is quickly used up. I am so fortunate to be supported by a family that not only has the financial resources to pay for rehab when those "covered" visits are depleted, but one that can provide me with the transportation that I need to get to rehab. If this were not the case, as it is for countless others, I would've been lying in bed all day, every day, and never would be able to function as independently as I do now.

It disturbs me that TBI is the number one injury facing returning veterans of the Iraq and Afghanistan Wars, and many veterans face a system ill-equipped for TBI. Since TBI often goes undiagnosed, many of these afflicted veterans receive no timely diagnosis, let alone rehab, leaving families faced with the daunting task of caring for a veteran without adequate support. I can only imagine how difficult it is for them to reintegrate into society after fighting a war, but to have to do so with a TBI is mind-boggling.

My physical and emotional recovery progressed to the point that I felt I could live on my own and integrate back into the world. I was itching to move out of my parents' house. It wasn't that I was on a short leash since I certainly wasn't going to be throwing crazy parties, but thankfully, that I had figured out how to keep myself clean and dress myself on my own without too much difficulty and was 25 years old and wanted to live on my own like anyone my age would.

In May of 2008 I began the transition. I was incredibly fortunate in the way this move came about. Since I still didn't have a license and the nearest city with any type of public transportation was Portsmouth, I knew it was the town I wanted to live in. An added benefit is that the location of The Krempels Center was along the bus route I would use. As anyone would be after acquiring a brain injury, I was a little nervous about moving out of my parents' house. As it happened—and not coincidently I imagine—my mom was looking to make a real estate investment in Portsmouth, NH through her business and she had my recently retired father doing some property hunting.

One day before picking me up at rehab, my Father saw some condos downtown that interested him. He contacted the listing agent, Bonnie Dridi, and set up a showing for that afternoon. When I got in his car, I was happy just to be sitting down after working hard in five hours of therapy when he asked, "Do you mind going to look at a piece of real estate with me?" I love my dad and know it's probably part of the reason he's successful, but when he gets his mind on accomplishing something he's like a pit-bull. Unless you have an electric taser or a fire hose shooting cold water, you can bet he's going to work until he is done with the task. I liked doing anything that broke up my routine of eating, sleeping, rehab, and doctors' appointments so I agreed, humoring myself that it mattered what I said.

We got to the condo building and met the agent, Bonnie, out front. As soon as we walked in the lobby, I was very impressed. The building was very new and nicely appointed. The unit we were looking at was on the third floor, a huge two bedroom with new appliances. I thought it was awesome. Bonnie saw the large scar on the front of my neck below my Adam's apple and asked, "Did you have a tracheotomy?" I was shocked that she knew what a tracheotomy was, let alone that it was the cause of my scar. I told her yes, and how I ended up needing it in the first place. "I had one of those too," she replied as she showed me that her neck was scarred too. I asked her what had happened to her and she told me about being involved in an incident in which she sustained not only a head injury, but also a spinal cord injury. I developed a great relationship with Bonnie because we could talk about the frustrations that people who had gone through similar type of traumas as we had, could understand. It gives me hope to see someone who has built a positive life after a big setback.

My father liked the property as well and my parents decided to capitalize on the recession-weakened housing market and buy the unit. Since it would be a while until the economy bounced back, my parents decided to hold the condo for a while and graciously allowed me to move in. The move took place in stages. At first I only stayed there with another person. Jeremiah, my mom, and a number of other people took a night to hang out with me and help me make the transition. I even started having Boomer stay over on occasion until eventually I was living on my own with Boomer.

As time passed I was more and more comfortable living on my own. Since The Krempels Center's three day a week schedule left me with two free days, I looked for a job in the financial field within walking distance of my new home. My first step in this very tedious and frustrating process was to set up some informational interviews. I set something up with seemingly every firm in town and I finally came upon a great opportunity. Merrill Lynch had an office in a building about 75 yards up the street from my door. I checked the Portsmouth office out online and saw an advisor's name I recognized, Rob Carrigg.

Rob was the then President of the board for The Krempels Center. I can't remember who set it up for me, but I had a meeting with him. He gave me some good ideas, but didn't need anyone at that time. I thanked him and left. A couple of days later, he contacted me to let me know he knew of another advisor, Steve Bricker, who could use someone and that I should call him. Steve is an awesome guy, a father of two, who I became pretty close to. He also had a really nice assistant named Christine who I worked side by side with. She was pregnant with her first child at the time and was awesome to work with because she has one of those personalities that put me in a good mood within an hour of getting to work. I enjoyed my three months at Merrill, but then I had a shift in my goals.

One day, when thinking about my future, I realized how lucky I had been to have made the recovery I did. Originally I had gotten into the financial services field to make as much money as possible. The money my dad sold his business for, and the support I was getting made me rethink my plans. Suddenly, money didn't have the same appeal to me and I wanted to share the wonderful opportunities I had and the lessons I'd learned with others. I had been helped by more than a few people in one important profession, and I decided I had a good chance of reaching my new goals as a Social Worker.

Attending Grad School was a scary proposition. It's tough for anyone, never mind for a brain injury survivor with a severe brain injury at that. I applied to UNH because of its proximity to Portsmouth and was delighted to learn of the school's great Masters of Social Work (MSW) program. Although I'd like to take all the credit, I know that my acceptance was due in large part to the letters of recommendation that were written for me by Dr. Michael Frass, Judith Ryan, and Steve Bricker. All three of them met me after my accident and only know the "new" Jim, so I guess he's a pretty good guy.

I took a summer class before starting in the fall of 2009, and was delighted to get an A, which gave me confidence heading into the year. I signed up for three classes which proved to be too stressful and I had to drop one, but I did well in both classes that I completed. I really enjoyed my classes and found my classmates compassionate about life and the subject.

The Future

I would love to be able to end my story describing how great I'm doing and that everything is fine, but that would be a lie. I'm still trying to get to the point where I don't have a desire to die. I used to think depression was a sign of weakness and strong people didn't get depressed, but now dealing with mental illness myself, I do think it is a chemical abnormality in the brain. I like to think of myself as a smart guy. I know I'm extremely fortunate and have everything that I need to survive. I have a lot of promise in my life. Even with all of that, I wake up most days wishing I hadn't. My real hope is to get over this depression and be o.k. with being alive.

When I sit back and try to analyze my whole life I am hurt by my incessant thinking and analysis. I have hard working parents who have been very successful, a brother who has his own serious health concerns but is battling, and a loving sister who moved back to the east coast to be closer to us. I just feel that one stupid decision on my part ruined everything. My parents should be focused on Andy's health, enjoying the time they have earned to relax; instead they're dealing with me being in and out of mental hospitals, struggling with eating disorders, and needing to be financially supported. After all, it was as recently as July, 2012 that I was in a residential treatment center for my trauma and eating disorder, so it continues.

Despite all of that, my physical recovery is going well and I continue to improve. I have finished my formal physical rehab, but continue to work out at Vision Fitness in Portsmouth, which has a huge selection of equipment and extremely friendly members. While not perfect, mentally I feel like my old self, which isn't always a good thing. I've reconnected with my close friends and have made some great new ones, particularly Jeremiah, who returned to Grad School at Duke to be a physician's assistant (PA) and my new roommate Chris, a hard working commercial real estate broker.

There is a notable absence of serious girlfriends in my story. I've always preferred to be single and "play the field." I don't want to sound pompous, but meeting girls was never tough for me, I just have a commitment phobia and always have. It's probably a good thing that I've gotten a lot of womanizing out of my system. I doubt that a 30 year old guy whose left side is impaired with no income and worst of all stands at only 5'4" makes me one of America's most desirable bachelors. I actually think I am ready to settle down a bit and someday get married, maybe even have children, if any girl would be crazy enough to fall in love with a goofy guy like me.

Another wonderful thing that I've started doing through The Krempels Center is Community Education in which members go to area schools and talk about brain injury and its prevention. I gain a tremendous amount of self worth in thinking that, perhaps through the telling of my story, I'll be able to prevent another kid from repeating my mistake. If this happens, in an odd way, I'll almost feel like this whole experience and its outcome has been positive.

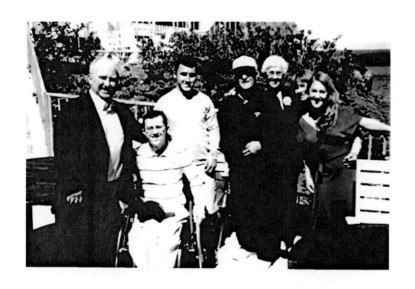

*My family and I at my sister's graduate school
graduation in June of 2012*

I Have a TBI---Now What?

To talk about the immediate phases of recovery from traumatic brain injury is very difficult for me. I have no clear recollection of the time from a couple of days prior to my car accident until my return to Spaulding in the ambulance with my Mother. I suppose this is my mind's way of protecting me from pain. Nothing from this lost period is particularly memorable, but those five weeks spent in an unresponsive vegetative state is where the groundwork of a new life was built. In a way it was fortunate that I hadn't matured into independent adulthood yet. Both my parents were—and are—very much involved in my life. Any period of time that anyone's decision making or ability to complete the requirements of daily living is compromised, it is vital to have someone entirely committed to their best interests in his or her corner, whether it's a spouse, parent or friend.

My parents made the decision that they wanted me to have aggressive rehab despite my bleak prognosis. Throughout my hospitalization, I had an advocate close by. Often this was an immediate family member in my room, but whether a relative or close friend, someone was never more than a phone call away. Obviously not everyone has the luxury of having self-employed family or multiple friends nearby, but this isn't an insurmountable barrier. If work constraints are the problem, most employers have policies allowing for leave time to care for a family member. Travel expenses can often be recouped through organizations, which a case or social worker at the hospital can help find. It was luck that I had many people immediately step in and take charge of my life for me. It's probably true for many that they don't have a large family or close friends nearby, but fortunately for individuals in this a situation it only takes one person to start a network. This person or group can be anyone or any organization that cares for you, from a relationship developed within churches, social clubs, or even volunteer activities. Post-TBI, I've developed relationships outside my long-standing friendships and family that may have worked if I had had no one step up for me.

Everyone needs a purpose

Whether the survivor is a parent, single or married, their role in society is turned upside down. Goals see immediate metamorphosis based on altered physical and cognitive abilities. It often seems like the world has continued to cruise along a smooth track while in your own life the brakes have been slammed on. This would leave anyone confused about where the hell they're going, not only a TBI survivor. You have to find a reason to go somewhere or life's treadmill is going to throw you off. This new direction often takes the form of purposes such as the responsibility of caring for a pet or making coffee in the morning, both of which proved huge in the early stages of my recovery. As life goes on this purpose will surely change. It could be that the recovery is proceeding greatly and allows parental duties to start again or the survivor can find gainful employment, but what matters is that this force creates the excitement to wake up in the morning, or simply a reason to do so. As the challenge of the purpose lessens and the excitement fades a new goal is needed in order to move on.

In recovery, continued skill creation requires further challenges. Of course, along with challenge comes the likely probability of failure so it's important for survivors and all people for that matter, to know their own stress and disappointment tolerances. My admittedly stubborn and inflexible personality has served me well in recovery while making me crazy, as evident in my story. Take it from me, set goals just high enough that hard work is required, but not too high that they always lead to failure. This isn't always an easy task and often requires the help of someone else. Ideally this person will be, or greatly resemble, the advocate for initial care. Now, you can't ignore reality. Problems occur, as they have and still do in my life when I ignore change and try to be someone I used to be. Ideally, anyone going through a life altering experience will realize that starting from scratch is the only option. It can be anything from a brain injury to a divorce, but a new beginning must be made. I've found that life's puzzle can't be put back together exactly as it looked before. Instead, each individual builds a new image, the best they can.

Acceptance doesn't mean giving up

After a trauma or disappointment in life, the fight or flight instinct kicks in. Flight usually takes the form of withdrawal from the world. This isolating behavior is certainly understandable but not helpful. Fighting to improve the situation either through rehabilitation or simply expressing one's opinion often leads to positive outcomes. However, fighting is exhausting and often leads to depression when gains seem to slow or stop completely. While I haven't reached this wonderful place yet, I know it exists from my wonderful association with The Krempels Center and its members: Reaching a place of being o.k. with the person you currently are, while working hard to reach goals every day, is the true acceptance I hope everyone reaches, including myself. Just like that son said to his father, for me, each day is a good day, just maybe with a few bad moments. If I just ride out those bad spots, yes, the whole is pretty good.

CPSIA information can be obtained at www.ICGtesting.com
Printed in the USA
LVOW06s1547131015

458070LV00001B/13/P

9 780988 537071